I0704823

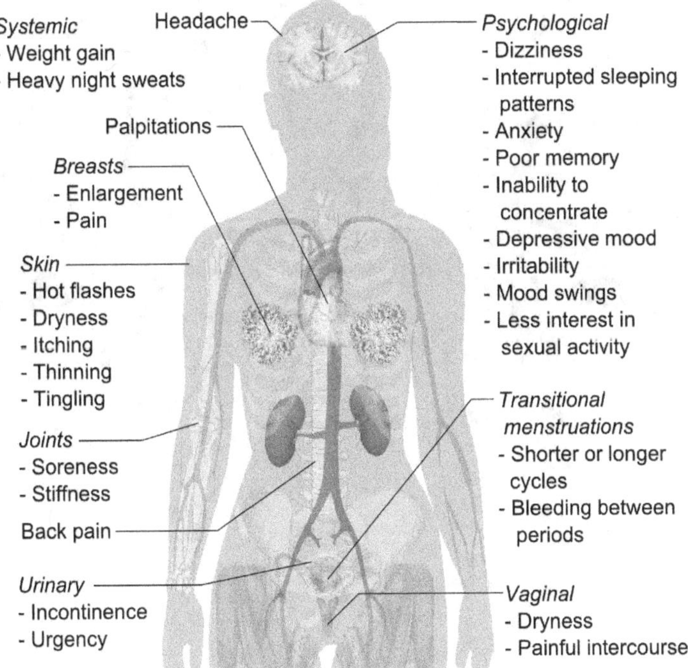

Symptoms of
Menopause
Headache
Systemic
- Weight gain
- Heavy night sweats
Palpitations
Breasts
- Enlargement
- Pain
Skin
- Hot flashes
- Dryness
- Itching
- Thinning
- Tingling
Joints
- Soreness
- Stiffness
Back pain
Urinary
- Incontinence
- Urgency
Psychological
- Dizziness
- Interrupted sleeping
  patterns
- Anxiety
- Poor memory
- Inability to
  concentrate
- Depressive mood
- Irritability
- Mood swings
- Less interest in
  sexual activity
Transitional
menstruations
- Shorter or longer
  cycles
- Bleeding between
  periods
Vaginal
- Dryness
- Painful intercourse

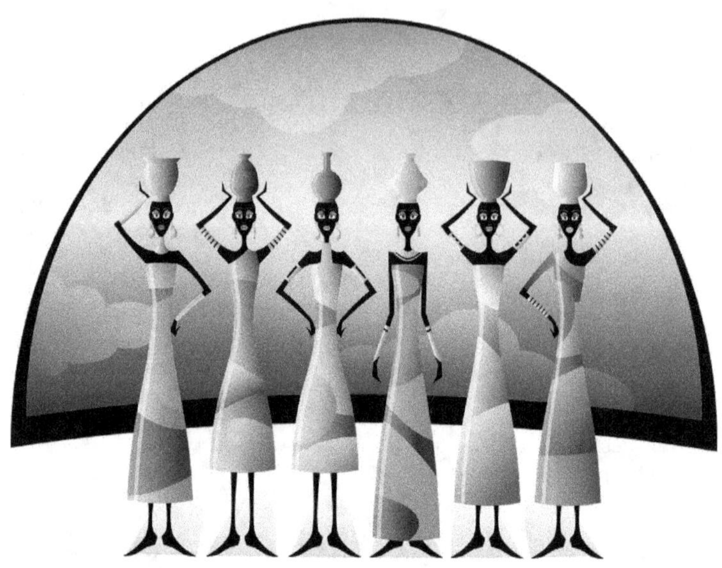

Men

O

Pause

BIBLE

Irritability

Itchy Skin

Joint Pain

Lack of motivation

Loss of confidence and self-esteem

Loss of Sex Drive

Memory Issues

Mood Swings

Muscle aches and pains

Muscle Tension

Nail Changes

Osteoporosis

Panic Disorder

Period Changes

Poor Concentration

Skin Changes

Sleep Issues

Stress Incontinence

Tingling extremities

What is menopause?

During menopause, a woman's oestrogen levels fall actually stopped having periods. This can often impact many areas of life both at work and at home.
Around three out of four of all women will experience some symptoms of a beast half of which will experience significant effects on the quality of their personal and social life with 75% of the women starting symptoms affecting them at work. In most cases symptoms continue for up to 7 years a one in 10 women for up to 12 years or more

The average age for the onset of menopause in the UK is 51 although symptoms can proceed to medicals by several years. An increasing number of women worldwide are now looking forward to living in at least a third of their lives in the post-menopausal state. With the great advances that have been made in the past 30 years in the synthesis of female hormones identical to those produced in nature to the benefit of large numbers of women, a dialogue is gradually emerging that is demystifying the issue.

Allergies

When your body contains frequently fluctuating levels of oestrogen this can lead to spikes in the production of histamine. This leads to your body becoming more sensitive to allergens than usual.

Symptoms
- Congestion due to seasonal allergies
- New food allergies
- Skin rashes
- Itching
- Swelling

Treatments
- Seek GP help
- Identity triggers of your allergies
- HRT
- Birth control hormone

Altered Skin Sensation

Experience numbness, pins and needles, prickling, itching or even the sensation of insects crawling over you.

Skin nerve functions may be affected by changes in the level of oestrogen in your body during perimenopause and menopause.

Symptoms
- Numbness
- Itching
- Dryness

Treatment
- Moisturizers and emollients
- Anti-histamines
- HRT
- Exercise
- Relaxation
- See your GP

Anxiety

A very common symptom that leaves you feeling stressed, tense, or fearful. Over the long term can lead to physical symptoms such as palpitations.

Symptoms
- Stressed
- Crying
- Stress incontinence

Treatment
- Exercise
- Limit sugar, salt, and processed foods
- Relaxation
- HRT
- Anti-depressants

Bladder Infections

Bladder infections or Urinary tract infections are very common and cause pain and burning while passing urine. Low oestrogen levels will
1. Make urethra delicate
2. Shorten urethra
3. The bladder may not fully empty
4. Bladder infection after sex

Symptoms
- Painful bladder
- Trouble fully emptying your bladder
- Urinary incontinence
- Night-time urination

Treatment
- Antibiotics
- HRT
- Vaginal Oestrogens
- See your GP

Vaginal Oestrogens
- May take at least three months to work
- No risk of breast cancer
- No risk of blood clots, stroke or heart disease
- Use for as long as you want
- Stopping treatment will bring back symptoms
- More vaginal discharge

Bladder Symptoms

Bladder issues include leaking, the need to go to the toilet at night, passing urine more often

Symptoms
- Pass urine more during the day and night
- Pain when you go to the loo
- The urgency to go increases
- Incontinence - stress
- Incontinence - urge
- Blood in urine

Treatment
- Talk to your GP
- Pelvic floor exercises
- Avoid alcohol and caffeine
- Stay hydrated
- Weight loss
- Bladder training
- HRT
- Vaginal Oestrogens

Bloating

This is a common symptom of perimenopause and menopause.

Symptoms
- Water retention
- Gas retention
- Body mass shifting

Treatments
- HRT
- Diet - eating patterns
- Exercise
- Reduce stress
- Quit smoking
- Talk with GP
- Understand your genetics

Body Odour

This is not uncommon during menopause when your body sweats more and a permanent change in odour is observed.

Symptoms
- The body reacts by sweating at lower temperatures
- Body reacts by shivering at higher temperatures
- Sweat more when stressed or anxious
- More bacteria in their sweat due to testosterone

Treatment
- HRT
- Fans and cooling sprays
- Cooling pillows
- Antiperspirants
- Extra strength deodorants
- Lose light cotton instead of synthetic
- Remove stress and anxiety

3 in 4 women experience hot flushes and nigh sweats related to menopause

Bowel Symptoms

These include bloating, wind, constipation, and indigestion. If you already have irritable bowels you may find your symptoms get worse.

Symptoms
- Heartburn
- Wind
- Reflux
- Diarrhoea

Treatment
- Diet and food diary
- HRT
- Stress Management
- Stay hydrated
- Stop smoking
- Avoid alcohol and caffeine
- Remove stress and anxiety

Brain Fog

Brain fog is a common symptom where you need to know how to recognize the signs.

Symptoms
- Difficulty concentrating
- Memory Loss
- Forgetfulness
- Difficulty recalling the right words
- Mood swings
- Depression
- Anxiety
- Sleep Issues

Treatment
- Sleep
- Exercise
- Diet
- Manage stress
- Find time to relax
- Develop coping strategies
- Keep brain activities
- HRT
- Testosterone
- Vitamin B6 and B12
- See your GP

73% of women experienced brain fog related to menopause

Breast Tenderness

Hormonal changes is the number one reason women have breast pain.

Symptoms
- Sore breasts 5 days before the menstrual period
- Breasts retain water
- Infection
- Injury
- Muscle strain
- Pregnancy

Treatments
- Check Bra
- Pain reliever
- Avoid caffeine
- Period Bra - larger bra than normal
- Reduce salt intake to limit water retention
- Relax and get enough sleep
- Yoga and meditation
- Wear a bra to bed - sports bra

Breast soreness

This is a common part of menopause where you get tenderness, burning, or soreness as they go through perimenopause and into menopause. Some will get a stabbing, sharp or throbbing pain.

Treatments
- Reduce salt intake
- Drink more water
- Avoid caffeine
- Low saturated fats
- Wear supportive bras
- Exercise regularly
- Apply a warm compress
- Avoid smoking
- Take a hot shower

See a Doctor if you have the following
- Change in size and shape of breasts
- Changes in skin texture
- Unexplained discharge
- Swelling or lump in the armpit
- A lump or abnormally firm area on the breast
- Persistent breast pain

Sore breasts are very common during the time leading up to menopause and the breasts may also change shape and size during that time.

Breathing Difficulties

Shortness of breath can be a symptom of menopause but you may have an underlying lung disease. Menopause transition can impact pre-existing lung diseases such as asthma or chronic obstructive airway disease (COAD).

Symptoms
- Anxiety
- Breathing issues
- Wheezing
- Coughing
- Chest pains
- Coughing up blood

Treatment
- Stay fit and active
- Stop smoking
- Singing to improve lung function
- HRT
- If acute or severe then see your GP

Brittle Nails

Lower oestrogen levels can lead to dehydration and leave your nails brittle and weak.

Symptoms
- Dry nails
- Brittle nails
- Nail infections
- Lack of energy
- Pale skin

Treatments
- Lack of iron - watercress, kale, meat
- Moisturiser
- Protect hands and nails
- Avoid acetone
- File nails
- Use a hardener for extra protection

Burning Mouth

Burning mouth syndrome can be linked to the loss of oestrogen. Other changes include dryness and changes in your sense of taste and smell.

The burning mouth can be linked to other medical conditions and lifestyle choices

Symptoms
- Mouth infections
- Allergies
- Acid Reflux
- Some medications
- Diabetes
- Underactive thyroid disease
- Drinking acidic drinks
- Over-brushing teeth
- Psychological conditions like anxiety, depression, and stress
- Lack of iron and vitamins B1, B2, B6, B9 and N12

Treatment
- Stop smoking
- Avoid certain foods
- HRT
- Talk with GP or dentist

Changes in taste and smell

Taste and smell can change with menopause. Falling oestrogen affects saliva, which can reduce or change our sensation of taste. Ageing can make these sensations less intense.

Symptoms
- Reduction in saliva flow
- Taste sensation is reduced or changed

Treatments
- Good dental hygiene
- Stay hydrated
- Chewing gum
- Artificial saliva pastilles and sprays
- Avoid alcohol and caffeine
- Stop smoking
- Apply lip balm
- HRT
- Visit your GP

Decreased libido

The loss of estrogen and testosterone may lead to changes in your body and sexual drive. You may not easily be aroused and may be less sensitive to touching and stroking which will lead to less interest in sex.

- Low libido
- Fewer sexual thoughts and fantasies
- Physical changes affect the enjoyment of sex

Treatments

- Medical treatments
- Lubricants
- Estrogen pills, creams, and vaginal rings
- Regular exercise
- Avoid or quit smoking
- Avoid alcohol and recreational drugs
- Avoid scented products
- Follow a nutritious diet
- Manage weight
- Pelvic floor exercises to increase vagina blood flow and strengthen vaginal muscles

Alternatives

- Acupuncture
- Aromatheraphy
- Yoga

Dental Issues

Gum disease and tooth decay may increase during menopause. A dry mouth can mean germs linger due to loss of oestrogen.

Symptoms
- Gum inflammation
- Bleeding gums
- Mouth and gum tenderness
- Receding gums
- Bad breath
- Bite issues
- Pain on chewing
- Loose teeth
- Infections

Treatments
- HRT
- Stop smoking
- Avoid sweet and acidic food and drink

Depression

Depression can be experienced at many varying degrees of intensity and duration which is a common symptom of menopause.

Symptoms
- Sad
- Low
- Losing interest in life
- Tearful
- Irritated
- Changes in appetite
- Disturbed sleep
- Fatigue
- Excessive or inappropriate guilt
- Feelings of worthlessness

Treatments
- Oestrogen is linked to serotonin levels
- Exercise
- Mindfulness
- Avoid alcohol
- HRT
- Antidepressants
- See your GP

Digestive problems

Lack of estrogen and progesterone during the menopause can slow down the process of food passing through your system and leads to water reabsorbed back into the bloodstream.

Symptoms
- Constipation
- Gas
- Bloating
- Stress
- Tummy ache
- Nausea

Treatments
- Take time to get up which will settle the hormone levels
- Breakfast to stabilize blood sugar levels
- Stay hydrated
- Chew your food thoroughly
- Probiotics

Difficulty Concentrating

This is very common and caused bu the direct effects of low oestrogen on brain function. Connected with low mood, anxiety, stress, and fatigue.

Symptoms
- Anxiety
- Depression
- Stressed
- Abnormal blood calcium levels
- Thyroid disease

Treatments
- Sleep
- Exercise
- Diet
- Manage stress
- Find time to relax
- Brain activities
- HRT
- Testosterone
- See a GP
- Low vitamin B6 and B12

Disrupted Sleep

Sleep can influence and be influenced by your health and other conditions as you move through menopause.

Symptoms
- Difficulty staying asleep
- Early morning wakening
- Less total sleep time
- Sleepiness/fatigue during the day
- Sleep apnoea
- Restless legs syndrome

Treatments
- Exercise
- Healthy eating
- Manage stress
- Intellectual stimulation
- Socially active
- HRT
- Yoga
- Massage
- Better sleep area
- Comfortable clothes
- Comfortable Bra if required
- Avoid screen time before bed
- Avoid caffeine before bed
- See your GP

Dizziness

Low oestrogen, increased anxiety, or swings in blood sugar. Consult your GP.

Symptoms
- Anxiety
- Stress
- Hot flushes
- Headaches and migraines
- Swings in blood sugar levels
- Vertigo
- Inner ear disease
- Fatigue
- Sinus infections

Treatments
- Stay hydrated
- Stand up slowly
- Maintain stable blood sugar
- Check inner ear
- Manage stress and anxiety
- HRT
- Consult your GP

Dry Eyes

Dry eyes can be a result of an oestrogen drop, leaving the eyes feeling gritty, itchy, and uncomfortable.
The dry feeling happens when you do not produce tears or are not effective due to a decrease in oestrogen.

Symptoms
- Stinging eyes
- Burning eyes
- Blurred Vision
- Eye irritation
-

Treatments
- Avoid irritants
- Limit screen time
- Lower your screen
- Artificial tears
- Keep hydrated
- HRT
- Visit your GP

Dry Mouth

Reduced oestrogen makes a dry mouth as salivary glands make less saliva which is important to keep the mouth and gums healthy.
Saliva protects your mouth against bacteria which means you are more prone to tooth decay, cavities, receding gums, and infections.

Symptoms
- Sore mouth
- Dry mouth
- Dry throat
- Dry lips
- Frequent thirst
- Hoarseness

Treatments
- Reduce stress/ Reduce anxiety
- Good dental hygiene
- Stay hydrated
- Chewing gum
- Artificial pastilles and sprays
- Avoid certain foods - very hot spicy or salty
- Avoid certain foods - sugary and acidic foods
- Avoid alcohol and caffeine
- Stop smoking
- Apply lip balm
- HRT
- Visit your GP

Electric Shocks

Lack of hormones may mean that the central nervous system starts to go haywire, signals may get crossed, amplified, short-circuited or distorted where you get the sensation of a shock or tingling all over your body.

Symptoms
- Shocks
- Tingling
- Headache

Treatments
- Plant-based oestrogen
    - Soya milk
    - Linseeds
    - Tofu
    - Pumpkin seeds
    - Sesame seeds
    - Sunflower seeds
- Exercise
- Reduce stress
- Yoga
- Deep breathing
- Meditation

Fatigue

Hormonal changes may lead to fatigue and tiredness. You may find it harder to sleep and may have night sweats.

Symptoms
- Physically exhausted
- Mentally exhausted
- Cutting out activities to cope
- Depression
- Anxiety
- Mood Swings

Treatments
- Low B12 and folic acid
- Low iron and anemia
- Nutritional deficiencies
- Sleep
- Excercise
- Nutrition
- Avoid alcohol
- HRT
- Relax

Fertility Issues

For most women fertility declines in their 30s, and further, the decline in their 40s as perimenopause begins. Early in the mid-50s the ovaries permanently stop releasing eggs.

Symptoms
- Irregular periods

Treatments
- Reduce stress
- Stop smoking
- Reduce alcohol
- Weight loss
- Have sex
- Seek GP advice

Forgetfulness

Issues with memory are a common source of worry, frustration, and stress caused by low oestrogen in the brain.

Symptoms
- Memory loss
- Depression
- Abnormal blood calcium levels
- Stress
- Low vitamin B6 and B12

Treatments
- Sleep
- Exercise
- Diet
- Memory aids
- Exercise your brain
- Testosterone
- See your GP

Gum Problems

Dry mouth can increase your risk of gum disease and cavities. In menopause you do not provide enough saliva to wash away oral bacteria, and germs can accumulate inside your mouth, raising your risk for gingivitis and tooth decay.

Symptoms
- Inflamed and receding gums
- Dry mouth
- Strange taste such as bitter or metallic

Treatments
- Full clean with a hygienist every three months
- HRT
- Avoid toothpaste with SLS
- Avoid acidic and spicy foods
- Alcohol can reduce strange metallic tastes
- See your Dentist / Doctor

Hair Changes

Hair can thin out all over, or from the crown or sides. The condition can cause hair to become brittle and make new hairs finer.

Symptoms
- Thinner hair
- Hair loss
- Low iron
- Stress
- Bald patches
- Losing hair in clumps
- Head itches and burns

Treatments
- Exercise
- Stop smoking
- Healthy diet
- Supplements
- Thickening sprays
- Wig
- Hair loss lotions
- Laser treatment
- Advice from GP

Hair Loss

Lack of hormone triggers an increase in androgens which shrink hair follicles which result in hair loss.

Symptoms
- Thinner hair
- Overall hair thinning
- Hair falls out in clumps
- Hair growth slower
- Hair to grow on face

Treatments
- Reduce stress
- Exercise
- Eat well - fatty acids
- Keep hydrated
- Avoid heat tools and styling
- Avoid hair dyes
- Use nourishing conditioner
- Wear a hat in the sun
- Wear swimming cap to avoid chlorine
- Talk to GP

Headaches and Migraines

Very common in women during menopause with severity and frequency related to loss of oestrogen.

Symptoms
- Migraines
- Flashing lights
- Floating spots
- Light sensitivity
- Nausea
- Pulsating pain

Treatments
- Yoga
- HRT
- Lower blood pressure
- Remove stress
- Wear blue light glasses
- Wear sunglasses
- Deep breathing

Headache and Migraine - tips

Many women get headaches or migraines caused by changes in their hormones.

Migraines are likely to develop in either the 2 days leading up to a period or the first 3 days during a period.

Tips
- Eat small frequent snacks to keep your blood sugar level increased
- Regular sleep pattern
- Avoid Stress
- Take regular exercise
- Relaxation strategies
- Migraine treatments
- Continuous contraceptive pills
- Hormone replacement therapy
- Oestrogen therapy

Heart Disease

Heart disease risk increases after menopause due to changes to blood vessels, cholesterol, and blood pressure.

Symptoms
- Heart Issues
- Raised cholesterol
- Diabetes
- Not enough exercise
- Obesity

Treatments
- Stop smoking
- HRT
- Exercise
- Look at diet
- Reduce alcohol intake
- Reduce cholesterol
- Reduce your blood pressure
- Heart disease and diabetes

Heart Palpitations

During menopause, it can be common to notice heart palpitations or irregular heartbeats feels like pondering and fluttering in the chest.

This is normal but it's always worth talking to your doctor.

Symptoms
- Medicine
- Fever
- Overactive thyroid gland
- Low blood sugar or low blood pressure
- Dehydration
- Intense exercise
- Low blood sugar

Treatments
- Manage anxiety
- Avoid alcohol and caffeine
- Prevent blood sugar dips
- HRT
- See the doctor

Hot flushes and night sweats

Irregular heartbeat

Irritability

Itchy Skin

Joint Pain

Loss of oestrogen can affect joints and connective tissue that 'glues' the skeleton together. This results in general muscle aches, pains, and stiffness.

Symptoms
- Inflammation
- Pain
- Swollen joints
- Stiff joints
- Painful joints

Treatments
- Weight control
- Stress reduction
- Quality sleep
- Yoga
- Painkillers
- Anti-inflammatory
- HRT
- See your GP

Lack of motivation

Loss of energy and negative thinking is common to feel this way and other symptoms change the way your body behaves.

Symptoms
- Anxiety
- Mood swings
- Depression
- Brain fog
- Memory issues
- Joint pains

Treatments
- HRT
- Deal with work issues
- Relaxation
- Exercise

Loss of confidence and self-esteem

Lots of triggers for loss of self-esteem. Some physical and some mental. It is a very common symptom.

Symptoms
- Anxiety
- Low mood
- Depression
- Brain Fog
- Memory Issues

Treatments
- HRT
- Work issues
- Relaxation
- Exercise
- Sleep

Loss of Sex Drive

Loss of sex drive is very common and is linked to vaginal symptoms like dryness and irritation, mood changes, and lower testosterone levels

Symptoms
- Sex painful
- Loss of arousal and desire
- Busy
- Stressed
- Tired
- Vaginal dryness

Treatments
- Speak to a sex and relationship therapist
- Maintain physical contact
- Make time and space to relax
- Make sex more pleasurable
- HRT
- Pelvic floor exercises
- Testosterone

Memory Issues

Mood Swings

Hormone swings with physical and mental symptoms of menopause can trigger mood swings.

Symptoms
- Low mood
- Anxiety
- Irritability
- Anger
- Tearful

Treatments
- Reduce alcohol
- Exercise
- Relaxation
- HRT
- Counselling
- Medication
- Talk to a GP

Muscle aches and pains

Oestrogen loss can affect joints and the connective tissue that holds your skeleton together. This leads to general muscle aches, pains, and stiffness.

Symptoms
- Muscles feel sore
- Fatigue
- Muscle aches

Treatments
- Exercise
- Weight control
- Posture and work environment
- Stress reduction
- Sleep
- Yoga
- Medication
- HRT
- See your GP

Muscle Tension

Nail Changes

Nails need moisture to keep healthy and lower oestrogen can lead to dehydration which can leave your nails brittle and weak.

Symptoms
- Dry nails
- Brittle nails

Treatments
- Use moisturizer
- Protect hands and nails
- Look after your nails
- Avoid acetone
- Patience to grow nail back
- Visit your GP

Osteoporosis

This is a condition where bones lose density, a change directly linked to a loss of oestrogen. No symptoms unless bones break.

Symptoms
- Change in posture
- Change in height

Treatments
- Get a DEXA scan
- Prevent fractures
- HRT
- Calcium and Vitamin D
- Regular exercise
- Stop smoking
- Drink less alcohol

Panic Disorder

Period Changes

Periods can become irregular, heavier, lighter, more or less frequent, and eventually, they stop completely.

Symptoms
- Miss a period
- Lighter
- Heavier or longer
- More frequent
- Pass clots
- Experience flooding
- Just stop out of the blue
- Fibroids
- Polyps

Treatments
- Contraceptive Pill
- Tranexamic acid - make periods lighter
- Mefenamic acid - make bleeding lighter
- Progesterone Pill
- Mirena coil
- HRT
- Sequential HRT - monthly bleed
- See your GP

Poor Concentration

Skin Changes

Loss of oestrogen can change our skin during menopause.
This will lead to dry skin, wrinkles, acne, and facial hair.
Skin will be more delicate and prone to bruising.

Symptoms
- skin drier and more sensitive
- Thinner and prone to damage and bruising
- More wrinkles
- Longer healing
- Acne
- Hairs appear on the face

Treatments
- Moisturise skin twice a day
- Protect skin from sun
- Try to stop smoking
- Avoid soap which dries skin
- Keep hydrated
- Pluck extra hairs
- HRT
-
- See your GP

Sleep Issues

Sleep issues are common and can be linked to aging. Poor sleep might be linked to hormone changes but physical issues at the moment can contribute as well

Symptoms
- Night sweats
- Joint pains
- Anxiety
- Low mood
- Depression
- Headaches

Treatments
- Reduce alcohol
- Reduce caffeine
- Solve chronic pain
- Lower your weight
- Avoid heavy or spicy foods
- Stop smoking
- Manage stress
- Manage sleep environment
- HRT
- See your GP

Stress Incontinence

Symptoms
Treatments

Tingling extremities

Symptoms
Treatments

Vaginal Dryness, itching, and irritation

Vaginal dryness, itching, and irritation are widespread menopause symptoms that impact over a third of menopausal women.

Symptoms
- Pain in the vagina
- Prickliness
- Yeast Infections
- Dryness

Treatments
- HRT
- Lubricants
- Vaginal moisturizers
- Avoid perfume products when bathing
- Soap-free wash
- Vaginal Oestrogens
- Vaginal laser treatment
- See your GP

Weight Gain

Weight gain can be linked directly to the menopause or can be caused by the effects of other symptoms, such as fatigue which leads to less activity.

Symptoms
- Slow weight gain
- Redistribution of fat from thighs to your middle
- Changes in appetite due to falling oestrogen
- Loss of muscle mass as we get older
- Tired
- Stressed
- Low mood

Treatments
- Fewer calories
- More exercise
- Time management
- Diet
- HRT
- See your GP

Hot flushes/flashes

During the menopausal transition, ovaries work less effectively and the production of estrogen and progesterone declines over time. This causes hot flashes and HRT steadies the levels of estrogen and progesterone in the body.

Seek GP help
Seek chemist advice
If hot flashes affect daily activities or sleep, Seek HELP

During a hot flash, you may have
- Sudden warmth spread through the chest, neck, and face
- Flushed appearance with red blotchy skin
- Rapid heartbeat
- Perspiration on the upper body
- The chilled feeling after a hot flash
- Feeling of anxiety

The frequency and intensity last at most no more than five minutes.

Risk Factors
- Smoking - more likely
- Obesity - higher frequency if high BMI
- Race - Black women get more hot flashes

Night Sweats

Night sweats are common in menopause, perimenopause, pregnancy, and during the menstrual cycle.

Menopause - very common cause
Idiopathic - body produces too much sweat
Infections - body trying to fight off infections
Cancers - most common is lymphoma
Medications - antidepressants can lead to night sweats
Hypoglycemia - Low Blood Sugar
Hormone disorders - several hormone disorders
Neurologic conditions - may lead to night sweats

Irregular periods

Irregular periods can happen around your 40s which could be Perimenopause.

This stage can last around four years on average and is due to fluctuations in hormones as you are running out of eggs in your ovaries. Estrogen levels drop and you have irregular menstrual cycles. You might get weight gain, hot flashes, trouble sleeping, vaginal dryness, mood changes, and depression

Permimenopause ends with the menopause at which point you have not had a period for 12 months.

Keep a menstrual diary which will gibe your OBGYN or GP an insight into what your body is doing and for how long.
Check abnormal uterine bleeding - amount of blood, frequency of bleeding and length of bleeding

Treatments
- Birth control pills
- Antidepressants
- Multi-Vitamins
- Meditation
- Exercise
- Relax

Mood swings

Some women have mood swings, anxiety and depression.

Drops in estrogen may affect how the body manages serotonin and norepinephrine, two substances that may have links to depression.

Lower levels of estrogen have links to irritability, fatigue, stress, forgetfulness, anxiety, and difficulty concentrating.

- Depression - Yoga, Anti-Depressants
- Anxiety - Yoga
- Low Mood - HRT, Omega-3, Diet rich in protein
- Irritability - Yoga
- Brain Fog - Exercise, Yoga and breathing

Vaginal dryness

Vaginal tissues become thinner and more easily irritated - resulting from the natural decline in your body's estrogen levels during menopause.

Symptoms
- Itchiness
- Irritation
- Painful sex

Top Tips to treat
- Avoid bubble baths, scented soaps, and lotions
- Try lubricants before sex
- Neutral creams to treat skin irritation in the vaginal area
- Topical hormone treatments to the vaginal area
- Take HRT
- Try medication such as Senshio

Treating these symptoms or preventing them can improve your quality of life and maintain comfortable intimacy.

Male Menopause

Low testosterone is a real issue for men as the decline in testosterone is a slower process. As men get older and changes in the function of the testes may occur as early as 45-50 and dramatically after the age of 70 in some men.

Symptoms
- Fatigue
- Weakness
- Depression
- Sexual problems
- Loss of interest in sex

Treatments
- Diet
- Exercise program
- Medications
- Antidepressants
- HRT

Partner Help

Partners are critical support during menopause
- Do not stress your partner about sex
- Talk about the symptoms
- Give the required space
- Understanding
- Listening
- Learning

Understand symptoms and impact
- Anxiety and depression
- Diminished sex drive
- Irritation, fatigue, and headaches
- Weight gain
- Hot flashes
- Sexual discomfort
- Vaginal dryness
- Mood swings

Support
- Mutually gratifying options for a change in sex life
- Give each other space
- Research treatment options
- Talk it out
- A new chapter of life

Mental health first aid

Algee action plan - A.L.G.E.E

Assess for risk of suicide or harm
Listen non-judgementally
Give re-assurance and information
Encourage appropriate professional help
Encourage self-help and other support strategies

Appendix

British Menopause Society
National Institute for Health and Care Excellence

British Menopause society Thebms.org.uk

Menopausematters.co.uk

Daisynetwork.org.uk

Healthtalk.org

Theros.org.uk

General Tips

Diet choices make time to notice how you feel after eating do you need to change your food choices

Exercise and to raise your heart rate daily listen to watch your body needs are made time to recover

Friendships many women withdraw from social interaction now is the time to make time for your trusted friends

Hydration is needed to help all your body systems work effectively, especially if having hot flushes

Incontinence too many women suffer in silence and this is often easily treated please consult your doctor

Joint pain keep moving stretch consider calcium and magnesium and soaking in Epsom salt bath

Keep talking it's too easy to become isolated and feel alone book chatting directly with friends

Night sweat and hot flushes identify your triggers e.g. alcohol caffeine and spicy food

Osteoporosis can be identified by a DEXA scan consider calcium vitamin di exercise and avoid alcohol and smoking

Peri menopause the stage leading up to menopause when oestrogen and progesterone levels begin to decline

Treatment you have choices for example doctor complimentary lifestyle choices coaching or mentoring

Unity tract infections drink lots of water possibly cranberry juice and see your doctor

Vagina or changes often highly treatable see a doctor and ask about localised oestrogen

Wait how we ate before menopause may need to change slightly to maintain a healthy weight

Yoga can be great for building pelvic core strength relaxation and getting some well-deserved time out

One down for 1 to 2 hours before bedtime journalling your gratitude and priorities for the next day

Myths of menopause

It's all about hot flushes
Hot flushes and night sweats are common symptoms of the menopause. Other symptoms such as vaginal dryness in continents reduce bone density weight gain reduce libido headaches hair sitting palpitations joint stiffness aches and pains and recurrent UTIs are some of the other symptoms that can affect women before during and after menopause

All symptoms are physical
Psychological symptoms such as low mood anxiety and panic attacks irritability feeling depressed difficulty concentrating and a feeling of aggression are all common in Perry menopausal and menopausal women. It is important to tell your doctor if you experience any of the symptoms so that they can offer you the right support and treatment

Menopause begins at 50
For most women menopause. Between the ages of 45 and 55 with an average age of 51 but symptoms can persist for several years.

Menopause Facts

There are many successful treatments
Optimising your lifestyle can have significant benefits
during menopause. Maintaining or achieving a healthy
weight, drinking alcohol in moderation, not smoking and
minimizing stress.
Getting adequate sleep and relaxation meditation yoga
can improve menopausal symptoms. Hot flashes can be
reduced by wearing light natural fabric clothing and
keeping the bedroom cool at night please discuss your
symptoms with your GP who may suggest that you
consider HRT or other prescription medications they
may also recommend CBT for symptoms of low mood.

Every woman has different symptoms. Each woman's
experience of menopause can be very different. Often
due to a lack of education about menopause women
may not be aware and may be unprepared when
symptoms present themselves. Most women would
experience some symptoms for the duration of the
severity of the symptoms fairies from woman to woman.

Remember every woman goes through menopause be
kind to yourself and don't struggle If you have troubling
symptoms speak to your GP for advice and support.

Menopause and employers

A key symptom of menopause is night sweats which could lead to a lack of sleep and fatigue. Ensure you are flexible with your employee's needs by allowing homework of them to be flexible with their working hours 3 out of 5 working women experiencing menopause symptoms say it has a negative impact on them at work.

Supporting and creating a positive environment between an employer and someone affected by menopause can help prevent the person from
- Lose confidence in skills and abilities
- Feeling the need to take time off work and hiding reasons
- Increased mental health conditions
- Leaving their job
- Discrimination

Employers should make sure they have steps, procedures and support in place to help staff affected by the menopause.
If an employee is treated less favorably because of their menopause symptoms, this could be discrimination if related to a protected characteristic, for example,

- Age
- Disability
- Gender reassignment
- Sex

Physical symptoms

Hot flushes / Night sweats
Insomnia / Disrupted sleep
Joint pain
Muscle ache
Osteoporosis brittle bones
Palpitations / Irregular heartbeat
Headaches / Dizzy spells
Nausea and digestive issues
Bloating
Weight gain at amino middle
Dry skin, hair loss, brittle nails
Breast pain/soreness
Vagina dryness
Urinary frequency
Burning mouth
Dental problems - Gum Problems
Irregular periods
Mood swings
Decreased libido
Digestive problems
Electric shocks
Aches and pains
An urgent or regular need to urinate
Irregular or very heavy periods
Poor concentration memory issues and inability to think
Cardiovascular disease CVD
Tingling extremities
Itchy skin
Fatigue
Anxiety
Stress incontinence
Brittle nails
Allergies
Body odour
Irritability
Depression
Panic disorder

Mental symptoms

Anxiety
Panic disorder
Mood swings
Depression
Difficulty concentrating
Brain fog
Memory loss
Word finding difficulty
Lots of self-confidence

PAGE LEFT BLANK FOR NOTES

PAGE LEFT BLANK FOR NOTES

PAGE LEFT BLANK FOR NOTES

PAGE LEFT BLANK FOR NOTES

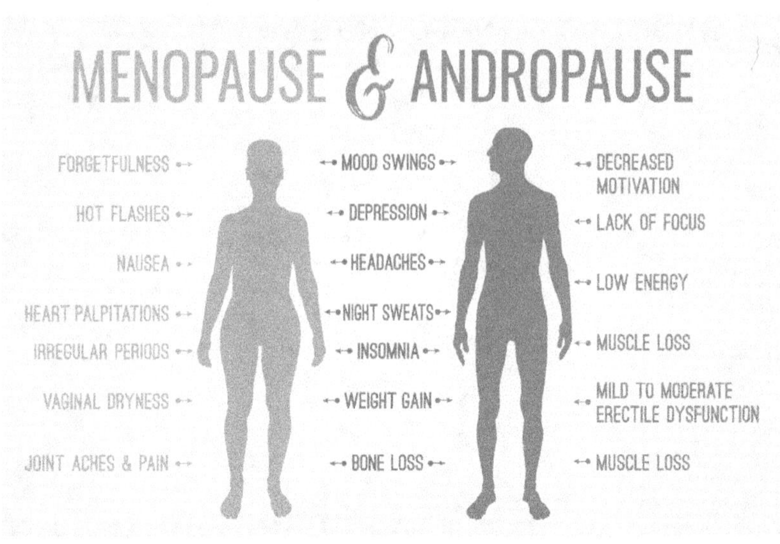

MENOPAUSE & ANDROPAUSE
FORGETFULNESS
HOT FLASHES
NAUSEA
HEART PALPITATIONS
IRREGULAR PERIODS
VAGINAL DRYNESS
JOINT ACHES & PAIN
MOOD SWINGS
DEPRESSION
HEADACHES
NIGHT SWEATS
INSOMNIA
WEIGHT GAIN
BONE LOSS
DECREASED MOTIVATION
LACK OF FOCUS
LOW ENERGY
MUSCLE LOSS
MILD TO MODERATE ERECTILE DYSFUNCTION
MUSCLE LOSS

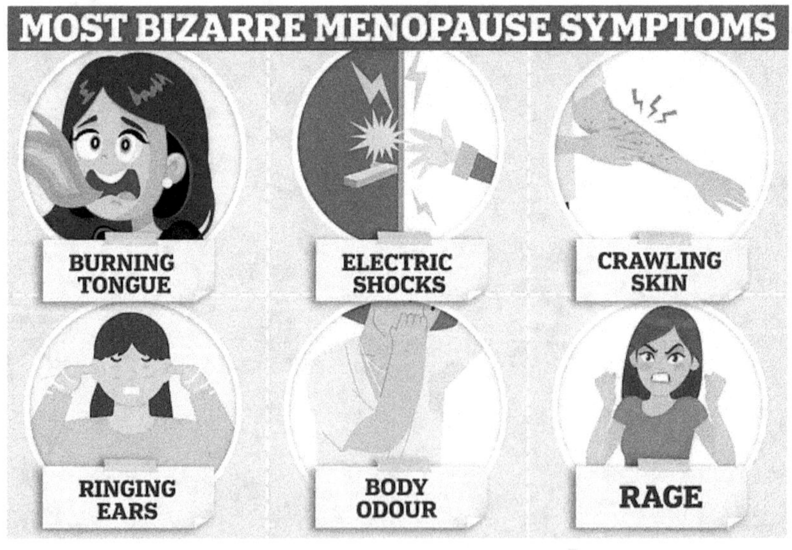

MOST BIZARRE MENOPAUSE SYMPTOMS
BURNING TONGUE
ELECTRIC SHOCKS
CRAWLING SKIN
RINGING EARS
BODY ODOUR
RAGE

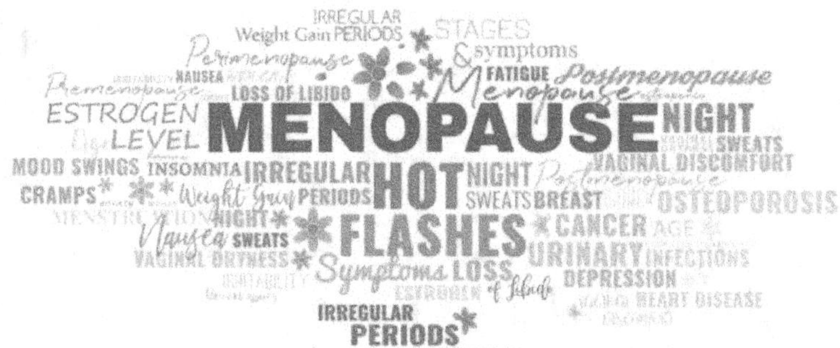

How Does Menopause Affect The Body?

Information for GPs and health professionals

National survey – The results

In May 2016, a survey conducted by Ipsos MORI on behalf of the British Menopause Society (BMS), has revealed that one in two women in Great Britain (aged 45-65 who past ten years) go through the menopause without consulting a healthcare professional. This is despite women surveyed reporting on average seven different symptoms and 42% saying their symptoms were worse or much worse than expected.

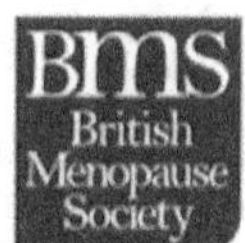

50%
of women **aged 45-65** who have currently experienced the menopause in the past 10 years, **had not consulted a heathcare professional** about their menopause symptoms.

This despite women reporting on **average seven symptoms** and **42% feeling their menopause symptoms** were worse or much worse than they suspected.

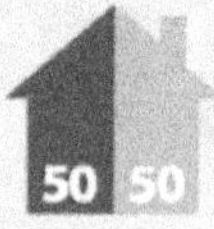

50% of women said their menopause symptoms had impacted their home life.

Many experienced symptoms they did not expect, including:

22% unexpected sleeping problems/ insomnia

20% difficulty with memory/ concentration

18% experienced unexpected achy joints

More than a third

said their menopause had impacted their work life.

79% of women surveyed experienced hot flushes and

70% experienced night sweats

36% women said their menopause symptoms impacted their social life

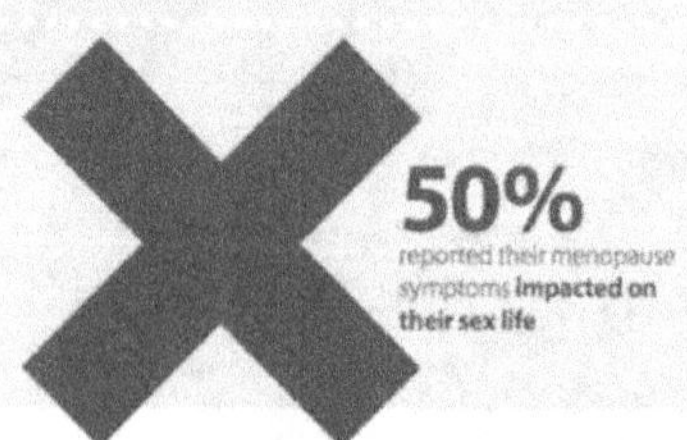

50% reported their menopause symptoms **impacted on their sex life**

For further details – please visit

www.thebms.org.uk or telephone **01628 890 199**

www.womens-health-concern.org
Reg Charity No: 279651
Company Reg No: 1432023

www.thebms.org.uk
Reg Charity No: 1015144
Company Reg No: 02759439

March 2017

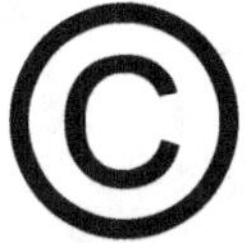

Copyright 2022 Nov MMM

www.ingramcontent.com/pod-product-compliance
Lightning Source LLC
Chambersburg PA
CBHW050817250726
48653CB00006B/2276